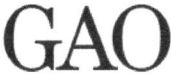

United States Government Accountability Office

Report to Congressional Committees

I0426175

June 2012

VETERANS' HEALTH CARE BUDGET

Transparency and Reliability of Some Estimates Supporting President's Request Could Be Improved

To access this report electronically, scan this QR Code.

Don't have a QR code reader? Several are available for free online.

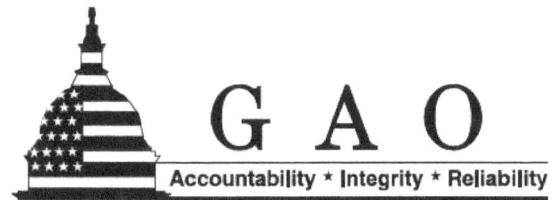

GAO

Accountability * Integrity * Reliability

GAO-12-689

GAO
Accountability * Integrity * Reliability
Highlights

Highlights of GAO-12-689, a report to congressional committees

VETERANS' HEALTH CARE BUDGET

Transparency and Reliability of Some Estimates Supporting President's Request Could Be Improved

Why GAO Did This Study

The Veterans Health Care Budget Reform and Transparency Act of 2009 requires GAO to report on the President's annual budget request to Congress for VA health care services. GAO's previous work found that VA's NRM spending exceeded its estimates in recent years and that some of VA's estimates of savings from operational improvements lacked analytical support or were flawed.

Building on GAO's past work and the President's most recent request for VA health care, this report examines (1) key changes to the fiscal year 2013 budget request compared to the 2013 advance appropriations request, and certain aspects of the fiscal year 2014 advance appropriation request and supporting estimates; and (2) whether the issues GAO identified regarding NRM and operational improvements continue in the estimates for the most recent request. GAO reviewed the President's budget request, VA's budget justification, and VA data. GAO interviewed VA officials and staff from the Office of Management and Budget.

What GAO Recommends

GAO recommends that VA state in its budget justification whether the estimates for initiatives include funding for ongoing services and whether its advance appropriations request reflects funding that may be required if initiatives are continued. GAO also recommends that VA's NRM estimates fully account for the long-standing pattern of medical facilities spending more on NRM than originally expected. VA concurred except for the recommendation on advance appropriations, which GAO believes is needed to improve transparency.

View GAO-12-689. For more information, contact Randall B. Williamson at (202) 512-7114 or williamsonr@gao.gov or Melissa Emrey-Arras at (617) 788-0534 or emreyarrasm@gao.gov.

What GAO Found

The President's fiscal year 2013 budget request for the Department of Veterans Affairs' (VA) health care services was $165 million more than the earlier advance appropriations request for the same year. This request reflected a $2 billion increase for initiatives and a $2.1 billion decrease for ongoing health care services, for a net decrease of $110 million in expected obligations. This decrease partially offset a decline in anticipated resources available to VA of $275 million, resulting in the net increase in the President's request of $165 million. Two of the three factors that accounted for most of these changes were not transparent. First, VA used a new reporting approach for initiatives that combined both funding for initiatives and for certain ongoing health care services in its initiatives estimate. Previously, VA had reported only funding it identified for initiatives during that year. This new reporting approach resulted in an increase in VA's initiatives estimate and a commensurate decrease in VA's ongoing services estimate. VA officials told GAO that this change was made to be more transparent about the total funding needed for initiatives. However, because VA did not disclose this change in its budget justification, VA has not made it transparent that its initiatives estimate is greater and its ongoing health care services estimate is lower than they would have been using VA's past approach. Second, VA included additional funding in its initiatives estimate, in part, to fund initiatives that were not identified in the fiscal year 2013 advance appropriations request. VA also did not make transparent in its budget justifications that some initiatives identified in its fiscal years 2013 and 2014 advance appropriations requests may require additional funding if the initiatives are continued. The lack of transparency regarding VA's estimates for initiatives and ongoing health care services results in unclear information for congressional deliberation.

The issues GAO previously identified related to NRM (non-recurring maintenance), such as renovations and other improvements of VA medical facilities, and operational improvements remain. VA's fiscal year 2013 estimate for NRM—$710 million—does not appear to correct for the long-standing pattern where VA's NRM spending exceeds VA's NRM estimates. For example, in fiscal year 2011 VA spent about $2 billion for NRM, which was $867 million more than estimated. According to VA officials, this pattern has occurred because VA medical facilities have spent more funds on NRM projects that were originally expected to be spent on other activities—such as utilities, grounds maintenance, and janitorial services—which is consistent with VA's authority to allocate its appropriations. When GAO asked if the fiscal year 2013 estimate addressed the historical discrepancies between estimated and actual NRM spending, VA officials said that all information was considered in developing the estimate. However, they noted that the final estimate was a policy decision and did not say specifically whether these discrepancies were addressed. Regarding operational improvements, VA estimated savings for fiscal year 2013 using the same methodologies it used in the past, some of which GAO previously found lacked analytical support or were flawed. GAO previously recommended that VA develop a sound methodology for estimating savings from its operational improvements, which according to officials, VA is addressing for future estimates. Until these issues are addressed, VA's estimates of NRM and operational improvements may not be reliable and are of limited use for decision makers.

_____ **United States Government Accountability Office**

Contents

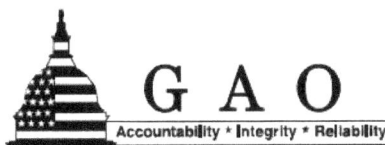

June 11, 2012

Congressional Committees

The Department of Veterans Affairs (VA) operates one of the largest health care delivery systems in the nation. VA provides a range of health care services for eligible veterans, including primary care, inpatient and outpatient surgery, prosthetics, mental health services, prescription drugs, and nursing home care.[1] In fiscal year 2011, VA served about 6.2 million patients and spent $51.4 billion on health care services. Unlike most other agencies, VA receives advance appropriations for health care in addition to annual appropriations.[2] In preparation for the appropriations process, therefore, VA develops an annual estimate of the resources needed to provide its health care services for 2 fiscal years. This budget estimate is reviewed through successively higher levels within the agency and revised until consolidated into a departmentwide annual budget estimate that is submitted to the Office of Management and Budget (OMB) for review and consideration. OMB subsequently includes both an

---

[1]Eligibility is determined on the basis of service-connected disability, income, and other special statuses, such as former prisoners of war, and is used to determine priority for VA services. VA is required to provide a specified set of health care services, including hospital care, to eligible veterans. 38 U.S.C. §§ 1710(a)(1), (2), 1701(5), (6). VA is authorized to provide these health care services to other veterans not identified in these groups. 38 U.S.C. § 1710(a)(3). The population of veterans to whom VA is required to provide nursing home care is more limited than the population to whom VA is required to provide other health care services, although VA also makes nursing home care available to other veterans on a discretionary basis as resources permit. See 38 U.S.C. § 1710A. Requirements for VA health care services are effective in any fiscal year only to the extent and in the amount provided in advance in appropriations acts for such purposes. 38 U.S.C. § 1710(a)(4).

[2]The Veterans Health Care Budget Reform and Transparency Act of 2009 provided that VA's annual appropriations for health care also include advance appropriations that become available 1 fiscal year after the fiscal year for which the appropriations act was enacted. Pub. L. No. 111-81, § 3, 123 Stat. 2137, 2137–38 (2009), codified at 38 U.S.C. § 117. The act provided for advance appropriations for VA's Medical Services, Medical Support and Compliance, and Medical Facilities appropriations accounts and directed VA to include with information it provides Congress in connection with the annual appropriations process detailed estimates of funds needed to provide its health care services for the fiscal year for which advance appropriations are to be provided. For example, Congress provided annual appropriations for VA health care of about $51.2 billion for fiscal year 2012 and advance appropriations of $52.6 billion for fiscal year 2013. Pub. L. No. 112-10, div. B, title X, § 2015, 125 Stat. 38, 175 (2011); Pub. L. No. 112-74, div. H, title II, 125 Stat. 786, 1149-50 (2011).

appropriations request for VA health care services for 1 fiscal year and an advance appropriations request for the next fiscal year in the President's annual budget request, which is submitted to Congress in February of each year.[3]

In support of the President's request, VA prepares an annual budget justification for Congress. The budget justification provides Congress and stakeholders with estimates and other information that support the policies and spending decisions represented in the President's budget request, including information on what VA plans to achieve with the resources requested. In particular, VA's budget justification includes detailed information on estimates of funding needed for ongoing health care services and health-care-related initiatives proposed by the Secretary of VA and the President. As such, VA's budget justification is used to provide Congress and stakeholders with important information about agency priorities, as well as the implications of the requested amounts for VA's provision of health care services to veterans.

The development of VA's health care budget estimate is inherently complex, as assumptions and imperfect information are used to project the likely quantity and cost of the health care services VA expects to provide.[4] Most of these projections are made several years into the future based on data from the most recent fiscal year. As such, VA's budget estimate is prepared in the context of uncertainties about the future—not only about program needs, but also about future economic conditions, presidential policies, and congressional actions that may affect the funding needs in the year for which the request is made. Our prior work has highlighted some of the challenges VA has faced in obtaining sufficient data; making accurate calculations and realistic assumptions when formulating its budget estimate; and developing estimates for non-

---

[3]For example, the President's fiscal year 2013 budget request included a request for VA health care for fiscal year 2013 as well as an advance appropriations request for fiscal year 2014. Next February, the President may request different appropriations for fiscal year 2014, which, if enacted, would supersede the enacted fiscal year 2014 advance appropriations.

[4]See GAO, *VA Health Care: Challenges in Budget Formulation and Execution*, GAO-09-459T (Washington, D.C.: Mar. 12, 2009).

recurring maintenance (NRM),[5] which have been consistently lower than actual expenditures in recent years.[6] In a February 2012 report, we found that VA's estimated savings from some operational improvements—used to support the President's budget request for fiscal year 2012 and advance appropriations request for fiscal year 2013—lacked analytical support or were flawed.[7] We made a recommendation to improve VA's operational improvement estimates. VA concurred with the recommendation except for two real property initiatives where VA maintained that the savings estimates were not flawed.

The Veterans Health Care Budget Reform and Transparency Act of 2009 requires us to report on the President's annual budget request to Congress for VA health care services. The law requires that we report on our analysis within 120 days after the President's budget requests are submitted in 2011, 2012, and 2013. Our June 2011 report, in response to the act, noted that in recent years VA's spending for NRM exceeded the amounts identified in VA's budget justifications and reflected in the President's budget request. We also raised concerns that VA may have to make difficult trade-offs to manage within its fiscal years 2012 and 2013 resources if the estimated savings from operational improvements, such as proposed changes to purchasing and contracting, do not materialize.[8] Building upon our work from our June 2011 report and in light of the

---

[5]NRM funds are used for expansion, renovation, and infrastructure improvements of VA health care facilities that cost more than $25,000. Examples include upgrades to safety, security, and fire alarms; interior or exterior renovations; improving accessibility for patients with disabilities; improvements to the heating, ventilation, and air conditioning; and projects to improve the roads or grounds.

[6]For example, see GAO, *VA Health Care: Budget Formulation and Reporting on Budget Execution Need Improvement*, GAO-06-958 (Washington, D.C.: Sept. 20, 2006); and *VA Health Care: Long-Term Care Strategic Planning and Budgeting Need Improvement*, GAO-09-145 (Washington, D.C.: Jan. 23, 2009).

[7]Operational improvements are actions the agency plans to undertake to better manage VA's health care system in an effort to improve the delivery of care and lower costs. See GAO, *VA Health Care: Methodology for Estimates and Process for Tracking Savings Need Improvement*, GAO-12-305 (Washington, D.C.: Feb. 27, 2012).

[8]GAO, *Veterans' Health Care Budget Estimate: Changes Were Made in Developing the President's Budget Request for Fiscal Years 2012 and 2013*, GAO-11-622 (Washington, D.C.: June 14, 2011). In this report, we examined key changes VA identified that were made to its health care budget estimate to develop the President's budget request for fiscal year 2012, including the advance appropriations request for fiscal year 2013, and how various sources of funding and other factors informed that request.

President's most recent request for VA health care services, which includes fiscal year 2013 appropriations and advance appropriations for fiscal year 2014, this report examines: (1) key changes to the President's fiscal year 2013 budget request compared to the advance appropriations request for the same year, as well as certain aspects of the fiscal year 2014 advance appropriations request and supporting estimates; and (2) whether the issues we previously identified regarding NRM and operational improvements continue in the estimates that support the President's fiscal year 2013 budget request.

To examine key changes between the President's fiscal year 2013 budget request and last year's advance appropriations request for fiscal year 2013, we reviewed and analyzed each request as well as VA documents and data related to the estimates that support them. We interviewed VA officials and OMB staff to discuss the key reasons for any differences between the estimates used to support the two requests. Finally, we reviewed the budget justification supporting the President's fiscal year 2013 request in the context of whether it provided Congress relevant information that could have a significant impact on VA achieving its objectives, including what VA plans to achieve with the resources requested.[9] Specifically, we evaluated whether VA informed Congress in its budget justification about key changes that occurred between the President's fiscal year 2013 budget request and the earlier, advance appropriations request for that same year.

To examine whether the issues we previously identified regarding NRM and operational improvements continue in the estimates that support the President's fiscal year 2013 budget request for VA, we reviewed VA's budget justification that supports this request. We also reviewed VA documents and data that described and supported the amounts VA estimated for NRM and the savings from the operational improvements. We interviewed VA officials and OMB staff to discuss the methods VA used to develop these estimates as well as the consistent pattern in recent years in which VA's spending for NRM has exceeded its estimates. In addition, we assessed the amounts estimated for NRM and operational improvements in VA's budget justification in the context of federal

---

[9]The federal standards for internal control for information and communication, in part, refer to an agency's ability to provide relevant information to stakeholders. See GAO, *Standards for Internal Control in the Federal Government*, GAO/AIMD-00-21.3.1 (Washington, D.C.: November 1999).

standards of internal control for information and communication. Specifically, we evaluated whether VA provided Congress reliable information for making decisions based on VA's NRM and operational improvements estimates for fiscal year 2013.

To assess the reliability of VA's estimates, we obtained documents supporting these data and verified the consistency of the information in these documents. We confirmed that the estimates were reflected in the President's fiscal year 2013 budget request for VA health care services and VA's related budget justification. We also relied on our prior work to compare data and check for internal consistency and discussed these data with VA officials. We found the data reliable for the purposes of comparing the fiscal year 2013 President's budget request with the earlier, advance appropriations request for that year and for examining whether the issues we previously identified for NRM and operational improvements continued in the estimates that support the President's fiscal year 2013 year budget request.

We conducted this performance audit from December 2011 through June 2012 in accordance with generally accepted government auditing standards. Those standards require that we plan and perform the audit to obtain sufficient, appropriate evidence to provide a reasonable basis for our findings and conclusions based on our audit objectives. We believe that the evidence obtained provides a reasonable basis for our findings and conclusions based on our audit objectives.

Background

VA provides health care services to various veteran populations— including an aging veteran population and a growing number of younger veterans returning from the military operations in Afghanistan and Iraq. VA operates approximately 150 hospitals, 130 nursing homes, 800 outpatient clinics, as well as other facilities to provide care to veterans. In general, veterans must enroll in VA health care to receive VA's medical benefits package—a set of services that includes a full range of hospital and outpatient services, prescription drugs, and long-term care services provided in veterans' own homes and in other locations in the community.[10] VA also provides some services that are not part of its

---

[10]VA provides adult day care, respite care, and other noninstitutional long-term care services as part of the medical benefits package it provides to all enrolled veterans. See 38 U.S.C. §§ 1701(6)(E), 1710B; 38 C.F.R. § 17.38.

medical benefits package, such as long-term care provided in nursing homes.

VA develops a health care budget estimate each year of the resources needed to provide these services for 2 fiscal years. Typically, VA's Veterans Health Administration (VHA), which administers VA's health care program, starts to develop a health care budget estimate approximately 10 months before the President submits the budget request to Congress the following February. The budget estimate includes the total cost of providing health care services, including direct patient costs as well as costs associated with management, administration, and maintenance of facilities. VA develops most of its budget estimate for health care services using the Enrollee Health Care Projection Model (EHCPM).[11] VA uses other methods to develop the remaining parts of its budget estimate, that is, the costs of long-term care and other health care programs.[12]

VA's annual budget estimate for a fiscal year includes estimates of anticipated funding from several sources. These sources include new appropriations, which refer to the appropriations to be provided during the current annual appropriations process for the upcoming fiscal year, and with respect to advance appropriations, the next fiscal year. For example, VA estimated it needed $52.7 billion in new appropriations for fiscal year 2013 and $54.5 billion for fiscal year 2014. In addition to new appropriations, sources of funding include resources expected to be available from unobligated balances and collections and reimbursements

---

[11]See GAO, *VA Health Care: VA Uses a Projection Model to Develop Most of Its Health Care Budget Estimate to Inform the President's Budget Request*, GAO-11-205 (Washington, D.C.: Jan. 31, 2011). For fiscal years 2013 and 2014, VA used the EHCPM to estimate resources needed for 59 health care services. The estimates are based on three basic components: the projected number of veterans who will be enrolled in VA health care, the projected quantity of health care services enrollees are expected to use, and the projected unit cost of providing these services—unit costs are the costs to VA of providing a unit of services, such as a 30-day supply of a prescription or a day of care at a medical facility. The EHCPM makes these projections 3 or 4 years into the future for budget purposes based on data available from the most recent fiscal year. For example, in 2011, VA used data from fiscal year 2010 to develop its health care budget estimate for the fiscal year 2013 request and advance appropriations request for 2014.

[12]The estimates for these services are based on factors, such as recent data on the costs and the amount of care VA provided to veterans, VA's policy goals for providing such services, and projections of the number of users.

that VA anticipates it will receive in the fiscal year.[13] VA's collections include third-party payments from veterans' private health care insurance for the treatment of nonservice-connected conditions and veterans' copayments for outpatient medications. VA's reimbursements include amounts VA receives for services provided under service agreements with the Department of Defense (DOD).

VA's health care budget estimate informs the President's annual request for appropriations for VA health care services, which includes an advance appropriations request for these services. The budget estimate can change during each budget formulation cycle, due to the availability of updated data and the successively higher levels of review in VA and OMB before the President's budget request is submitted to Congress. The Secretary of VA considers the health care budget estimate developed by VHA when assessing resource requirements among competing interests within VA, and OMB considers overall resource needs and competing priorities of other agencies when deciding the level of funding requested for VA's health care services. VA prepares a budget justification that provides information supporting the policy and funding decisions in the President's budget request. In its budget justification, VA includes estimates related to the following:

- **Ongoing health care services**, which include acute care, rehabilitative care, mental health, long-term care, and other health care programs.[14]

- **Initiatives**, which are proposals by the Secretary of VA or by the President to provide, expand, or create new health care services.

---

[13]In addition to new appropriations that VA may receive from Congress as a result of the annual appropriations process, funding may also be available from unobligated balances of multiyear appropriations, which remain available for a fixed period of time in excess of 1 fiscal year. For example, VA's fiscal year 2012 appropriations provided that about $1.75 billion be available for 2 fiscal years. These funds may be carried over from fiscal year 2012 to fiscal year 2013 if they are not obligated by the end of fiscal year 2012. See Pub. L. No. 112-74, div. H, title II, § 227(b), 125 Stat. 786, 1159 (2011).

[14]Based on fiscal year 2011 data, the largest of VA's other services was the Civilian Health and Medical Program of the Department of Veterans Affairs, which provides health care coverage for the dependents and survivors of veterans who are, or were at the time of death, permanently and totally disabled from a service-connected disability, or who died in the line of duty or from a service-connected condition. See 38 U.S.C. § 1781.

Some of the proposed initiatives can be implemented within VA's existing authority, while other initiatives would require a change in law.

- **Operational improvements**, which are changes in the way VA manages its health care system to lower costs, such as changes to its purchasing and contracting strategies.

- **Collections and reimbursements**, which are resources VA expects to collect from health insurers of veterans who receive VA care for nonservice-connected conditions and other sources, such as veterans' copayments, and to receive as reimbursement of services provided to other government agencies or private or nonprofit entities.

VA Changed Estimates Supporting the Request, but Factors That Account for Most of the Changes Were Not Transparent

Request Increased $165 Million, Reflecting an Increase in Initiatives and a Decrease in Both Ongoing Services and Available Resources

The President's fiscal year 2013 budget request for VA health care services was $165 million more than the advance appropriations request for the same year. This increase came about as a result of changes in the estimates supporting the two requests. Specifically, the President's fiscal year 2013 request reflected an estimate of funding needed for initiatives that increased by $2 billion and an estimate for ongoing health care services that decreased by $2.1 billion, for a net decrease of $110 million. In addition, VA's estimate of anticipated resources from collections and reimbursements decreased by $275 million. This decline in anticipated resources was partially offset by the $110 million decrease in expected obligations, which resulted in the net increase in the President's request of $165 million.[15] (See table 1.)

Table 1: Comparison of the Estimates That Supported the President's Advance Appropriations Request and President's Budget Request and the Effect of Any Differences on the President's Budget Request, Fiscal Year 2013

(Dollars in millions)

Description	President's fiscal year 2013 advance appropriations request	President's fiscal year 2013 budget request	Effect of the difference in estimates on President's fiscal year 2013 budget request
Ongoing health care services[a]	$56,628	$54,523	($2,105)
Initiatives[b]	$1,346	$3,341	$1,995
Operational improvements	($1,284)	($1,284)	$0
Total obligations	**$56,690**	**$56,580**	**($110)**
Collections and reimbursements	($3,649)	($3,374)	$275
Unobligated balances	($500)	($500)	$0
Total appropriations	**$52,541**	**$52,706**	**$165**

Source: GAO analysis of VA's congressional budget justification for fiscal year 2013 and VA's congressional budget justification for fiscal year 2012—which supported the President's advance appropriations request for fiscal year 2013.

[a]Ongoing health care services include acute care, rehabilitative care, mental health, long-term care, and other health care programs.

[b]Initiatives include those that can be implemented within VA's existing authority and other initiatives that would require a change in law.

Three Factors Accounted for Most Changes to Supporting Estimates, but Two Were Not Transparent

Three factors accounted for most of the changes in the estimates that supported the President's fiscal year 2013 budget request when compared to the earlier, advance appropriations request; however, VA, in its budget justification, was not transparent about two of the factors. The three factors that accounted for the $2 billion increase in the initiatives estimate and the $2.1 billion decrease in the ongoing health care services estimate were: (1) a new approach in reporting the estimate for initiatives, (2) updated assumptions and data to estimate ongoing health care

[15]Anticipated collections for fiscal year 2013 decreased $325 million from the estimate provided with the advance appropriations request for that year; however, $50 million of this decrease was offset by an estimated increase in reimbursements in fiscal year 2013, compared to the estimate reflected in the advance appropriations request. The decrease in collections was due to many factors including VA using a new projection model for collections—rather than historical data—to inform the President's fiscal year 2013 request, fewer enrollees having comprehensive health insurance that VA can bill for services that VA provides, lower payment amounts from insurance companies, and aging enrollees which results in VA billing more Medigap policies rather than full health insurance policies.

services, and (3) additional funding needed for initiatives. The first factor—VA's new reporting approach—accounted for $1.2 billion of the increase in VA's initiatives estimate and a corresponding decrease in VA's ongoing health care services estimate. The second factor accounted for a $900 million decrease in VA's ongoing health care services estimate. This decrease was largely offset by the third key factor—an almost $800 million increase in additional funding for initiatives. (See table 2.)

Table 2: Key Factors That Accounted for Changes Made to VA's Estimates for Ongoing Health Care Services and Initiatives Supporting the President's Fiscal Year 2013 Budget Request

(Dollars in millions)

	Ongoing services estimate	Initiatives estimate
New reporting approach	($1,213)	$1,213
Updated data and assumptions for ongoing health care services	($892)	Not applicable
Additional funding for initiatives	Not applicable	$782
Total difference in estimates due to three key factors	**($2,105)**	**$1,995**

Source: GAO analysis of VA's congressional budget justification for fiscal year 2013 and VA's congressional budget justification for fiscal year 2012—which supported the President's advance appropriations request for fiscal year 2013.

A new approach in reporting the estimate for initiatives. VA used a new reporting approach for initiatives that combined both funding for initiatives and funding for certain ongoing health care services in its initiatives estimate, which increased VA's initiatives estimate and decreased VA's ongoing services estimate. In prior budget justifications, VA's estimated funding for initiatives only included funding identified for initiatives during that year while funding needs for all ongoing services were included in VA's estimate for ongoing health care services. However, VA, in its budget justification, did not disclose that it had used a new reporting approach for initiatives. OMB staff and VA officials told us that the reason for this change in reporting was to be more transparent about the total amount of funding needed to support VA's initiatives. Nevertheless, by not stating in its budget justification that it made this change, VA has not made it transparent that the estimate for initiatives is greater and the estimate for ongoing services is less than they would have been using VA's past reporting approach.

Updated data and assumptions to estimate ongoing health care services. As reported in its budget justification, VA used updated assumptions and data, which reduced VA's estimate for ongoing health care services. Specifically, the amount of funding needed to support health care services estimated by the EHCPM decreased because VA updated some

GAO-12-689 VA Health Care Budget

of the assumptions used in the EHCPM. For example, VA updated the EHCPM's assumption accounting for the pay freeze for civilian employees in fiscal years 2011 and 2012, which reduced the base salary of VA employees in future years. VA also used updated data to adjust the estimates produced by the EHCPM and the estimates for long-term care and other health care programs. Updated data for long-term care and other health care programs generally indicated that costs for these services would grow at a slower rate than the data used to support the President's fiscal year 2013 advance appropriations request indicated.

Additional funding for initiatives. According to VA's budget justification, as a result of the reduced estimate for ongoing health care services, VA increased the estimate of funding needed for its initiatives. This estimate of funding included funding for all initiatives for which funding was not requested in the fiscal year 2013 advance appropriations request and increased funding for some initiatives for which funding had been identified in the earlier request.[16] However, in its fiscal year 2013 budget justification, VA did not make it clear that part of the additional increase in its initiatives estimate occurred because VA's earlier estimate in support of the advance appropriations request did not include funding for all the initiatives the agency intended to continue. According to OMB staff, the purpose of the advance appropriations request is to provide assurance for the continuation of ongoing health care services and select initiatives that represent direct care to veterans. As a result, rather than including estimates of funding needed to support all initiatives in advance appropriations requests—including the fiscal year 2013 advance appropriations request and the fiscal year 2014 advance appropriations request—the funding needs for all initiatives are taken into account during the following budget formulation cycle. At that time, once updated data are available to produce revised estimates for ongoing health care services, VA and OMB assess the amount of likely resources available to fund initiatives in the context of overall budget constraints. However, VA did not state that some initiatives for which estimates were included in the fiscal years 2013 and 2014 advance appropriations requests would

---

[16]According to VA officials, VA's revised initiatives estimate also reflects the use of more current data, although this was not the primary reason for the increase in the initiatives estimate. For example, more recent data on the equipment and supplies and additional personnel costs associated with the activation of completed construction of new or replacement medical care facilities informed VA's fiscal year 2013 estimate for the activation initiative.

require additional funding if the initiatives were to be continued. (Table 3 indicates the difference in the fiscal year 2013 initiative estimates attributable to VA's new reporting approach versus additional funding.)

Table 3: Comparison of Differences in Estimates for Initiatives That Supported the President's Advance Appropriations Request and the President's Budget Request, Fiscal Year 2013

(Dollars in millions)

Initiatives and legislative proposals:	President's fiscal year 2013 advance appropriations request	President's fiscal year 2013 budget request	Difference due to new reporting approach	Difference due to additional funding for initiatives[a]
Activations	$344	$792	$83	$365
Agent Orange	$191	$191	$0	$0
Amyotrophic Lateral Sclerosis	$47	$47	$0	$0
Caregivers and Veteran Omnibus Health Services	$248	$278	$0	$30
DOD/VA Integrated Disability Evaluations System Enhancement	$19	$22	$0	$3
Indian Health Services	$57	$52	$0	($5)
Homelessness: Zero Homelessness	$460	$1,352	$678	$214
New Models of Patient-Centered Care	$0	$433	$354	$79
Expand Health Care Access for Veterans	$0	$120	$98	$22
Improve the Quality of Health Care while Reducing Costs	$0	$51	$0	$51
Establish World-Class Health Informatics Capability	$0	$10	$0	$10
Improving Veteran Mental Health[b]	Not applicable	$20	$0	$20
Legislative Proposals	($20)	($27)	$0	($7)
Total initiatives	**$1,346**	**$3,341**	**$1,213**	**$782**

Source: GAO analysis of VA's congressional budget justification for fiscal year 2013 and VA's congressional budget justification for fiscal year 2012—which supported the President's advance appropriations request for fiscal year 2013.

[a]According to VA officials, part of the difference in the initiative estimate is also due to revised estimates for each initiative based on more current data; however, officials stated that this was not a primary reason for the difference in the initiative estimate between the President's fiscal year 2013 budget request and the earlier advance appropriations request.

[b]The improving Veteran Mental Health initiative was not included in the fiscal year 2013 advance appropriations request.

VA's budget justification is used to provide Congress with relevant information for making decisions. The lack of transparency regarding the factors that changed VA's estimates for ongoing health care services and initiatives results in unclear information for congressional deliberation.

Past Issues in VA's Estimates for NRM and Operational Improvements Remain

Our analysis of the estimates supporting the President's fiscal year 2013 budget request found that VA's supporting estimates (1) do not address historical discrepancies between estimated and actual NRM spending and (2) lack analytical support for expected savings from some operational improvements.

Regarding NRM, VA's fiscal year 2013 estimate does not appear to correct for the long-standing pattern of VA's NRM spending exceeding its estimates and was based on a policy decision. In June 2011, we reported VA's spending on NRM exceeded the estimates reported in VA's budget justifications from fiscal years 2006 to 2010.[17] More recently, we found that in fiscal year 2011 VA spent about $2 billion for NRM, which was $867 million more than estimated (see fig. 1). According to VA officials, NRM spending has exceeded estimates of needed funding in recent years because VA medical facilities have spent more funds on NRM projects that were originally expected to be spent on other activities—such as utilities, grounds maintenance, and janitorial services. This spending is consistent with VA's authority to increase or decrease the amounts VA allocates from the Medical Facilities account for NRM and with congressional committee report language.[18] When we asked VA officials if the fiscal year 2013 estimate addressed the historical discrepancies between amounts estimated and actual spending, VA officials said that all information was considered in developing the estimate. However, VA officials noted that the amount requested was a policy decision and did not specifically say whether these discrepancies were addressed. This explanation suggests that VA has not changed the way in which it determines the final NRM estimate; as we previously reported VA lowered its fiscal year 2012 estimate due to a policy decision to fund other initiatives.[19] Because the fiscal year 2013 estimate of $710

---

[17]See GAO-11-622.

[18]See, e.g., S. Rep. No. 111-40 (2009), at 57; H.R. Rep. No. 111-188 (2009), at 43-44.

[19]See GAO-11-622.

million is significantly lower than past spending and lower than the estimate provided last year, it does not appear that medical facilities' spending was addressed. Furthermore, VA estimates that the NRM backlog for health care facilities—which reflects the total amount needed to address facility deficiencies—will remain over $9 billion in fiscal year 2013. As such, the NRM information provided in VA's budget justification may not be a reliable estimate of future spending for NRM.

Figure 1: Non-Recurring Maintenance (NRM) Estimates That Support the President's Budget Request and VA's NRM Spending, Fiscal Years 2006 to 2014

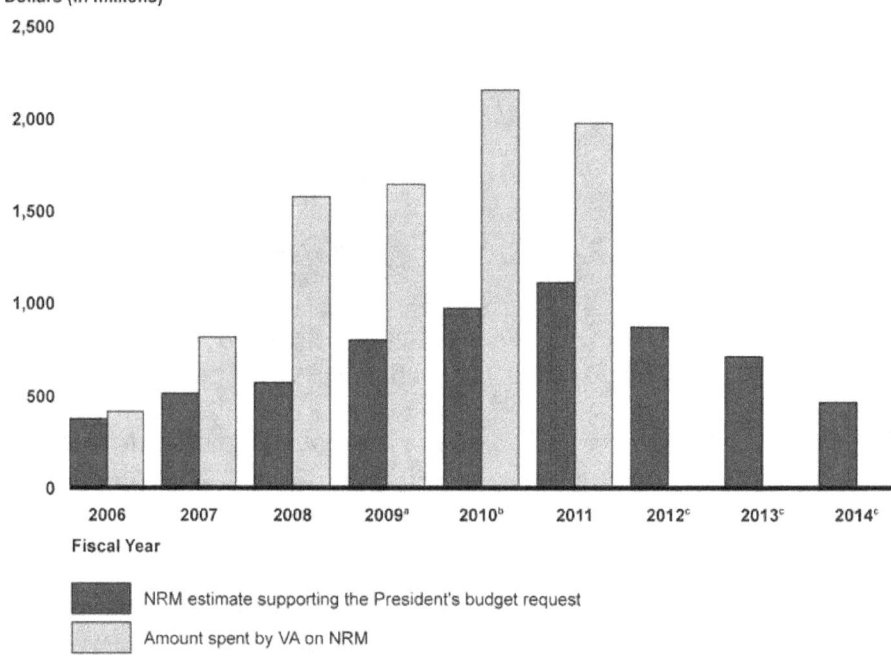

Source: GAO analysis of VA's congressional budget justifications for fiscal years 2006 through 2013.

Note: NRM spending reflects obligated amounts.

[a]VA was provided $1 billion for NRM—in addition to the fiscal year 2009 appropriations for the Medical Facilities account—as part of the American Recovery and Reinvestment Act of 2009 (Recovery Act). The Recovery Act funding was outside the scope of the President's fiscal year 2009 budget request. VA spent about $260 million of this Recovery Act funding on NRM in fiscal year 2009.

[b]The NRM amount reflected in the President's fiscal year 2010 budget request included $510 million from the Recovery Act. However, VA had about $740 million in Recovery Act funding available for fiscal year 2010, and VA spent all of the remaining Recovery Act funding in fiscal year 2010.

[c]Amounts spent not available for fiscal years 2012 through 2014.

Regarding operational improvements, VA estimated savings for fiscal year 2013 using the same methodologies it used in the past, some of which we recently reported lacked analytical support or were flawed.[20] The President's budget request for fiscal year 2013 reflected VA's estimate that it would save about $1.3 billion from the implementation of six operational improvements:

- *Changing rates*. Estimated savings from purchasing dialysis treatments and other care from civilian providers at Medicare rates instead of current community rates.

- *Acquisitions*. Estimated cost savings from changes to VA's purchasing and contracting strategies.

- *Fee Care*. Estimated saving from purchasing care from non-VA providers at lower rates.

- *Realigning clinical staff and resources*. Estimated savings by using less costly health care providers, such as licensed practical nurses instead of certain types of registered nurses.

- *Medical and administrative support*. Estimated savings from employing resources more efficiently.

- *VA real property*. Estimated saving from initiatives including repurposing vacant or underutilized buildings, decreasing energy costs, and changing procurement practices for building maintenance.

In a February 2012 report, we highlighted issues regarding VA's methodology for estimating savings from some operational improvements, including changes to VA real property, medical and administrative support activities, and the realignment of clinical staff and resources. We also recommended that VA develop a sound methodology for estimating savings from its operational improvements.[21] In response, VA concurred with the recommendation except for two real property initiatives where VA maintained that the savings estimates were not flawed. However, since our February report was issued after the release

---

[20]See GAO-12-305.

[21]We also recommended that VA develop a detailed process for tracking actual savings resulting from those improvements for which we identified concerns. See GAO-12-305.

GAO-12-689 VA Health Care Budget

of the President's budget request for fiscal year 2013, VA has not yet implemented our recommendations. VA officials told us during the course of our current review that the agency is taking steps to address deficiencies in the methodology used for estimating savings for some of its operational improvements. Without a sound methodology, VA runs the risk of falling short of its estimated savings, which may ultimately require VA to make difficult trade-offs to provide health care services with the available resources. We determined that the estimates for some of the operational improvements provided in VA's budget justification may not be reliable estimates of future savings and therefore are of limited use for decision makers.

Conclusions

VA's budget justification is intended to provide Congress with estimates of resource needs and what the agency plans to achieve with requested appropriations. Our work shows that changes in the way that VA estimates and reports its required resources are responsible for the increase in the President's fiscal year 2013 budget request for VA health care, when compared to last year's advance appropriations request for the same year. However, VA was not transparent in its budget justification about two of the factors that accounted for the change in VA's initiatives and ongoing health care services estimates. By neither disclosing that it used a new reporting approach for initiatives nor indicating that its advance appropriations requests did not include funding for continuing initiatives, VA did not provide Congress with information relevant to understanding these estimates.

In addition, VA may not have provided Congress reliable information with which to make decisions regarding VA's appropriations in regards to NRM and some operational improvements. VA's most recent NRM estimates do not appear to correct for the long-standing pattern where VA's NRM spending exceeds VA's NRM estimates. VA's estimates have not consistently accounted for additional spending by VA medical facilities. As a result, the NRM estimates may be unreliable, as they may continue to underestimate VA's future spending for NRM. Also, VA continued to use flawed methodologies we identified in our prior work to develop savings estimates for operational improvements. We continue to believe that VA should improve its methodology as we previously recommended. Until these issues are addressed, VA's estimates of NRM and operational improvements are of limited use for decision makers.

Recommendations for Executive Action

To improve the transparency and reliability of information presented in VA's congressional budget justifications that support the President's budget request for VA health care, we recommend the Secretary of VA take the following three actions:

- State in future budget justifications whether the estimates for initiatives include funding for ongoing health care services.

- State in future budget justifications whether the estimates for initiatives in support of the advance appropriations request reflect all the funding that may be required if all initiatives are to be continued.

- Reflect in future budget justifications estimates of annual resource needs for NRM that fully account for resources that VA medical facilities have consistently spent for this purpose.

Agency Comments and Our Evaluation

We provided a draft of this report to the Secretary of VA and the Acting Director of OMB for comment. In its written comments signed by the Chief of Staff and reprinted in appendix I, VA concurred with two of our three recommendations, but did not concur with our recommendation related to the estimates for initiatives that support VA's advance appropriations requests. In addition, VA stated in its comments that one aspect of our report is not accurate, that it disagrees with a second, and that it had concerns about a third. OMB staff provided a technical comment, which we incorporated.

VA concurred with our first recommendation regarding funding for ongoing health care services. VA noted that to implement this recommendation it will include in future budget justifications a narrative description stating whether the estimates for initiatives include funding for ongoing health care services. VA also concurred with our third recommendation regarding its estimates for NRM. VA noted that in order to implement this recommendation, VA will reflect in future budget justifications annual estimates of resources needed for NRM that are consistent with policy decisions and account for past spending on NRM.

VA did not concur with our second recommendation related to the estimates for initiatives that support VA's advance appropriations requests. VA stated that it did not concur because the recommendation is not consistent with its multiyear approach to budgeting for advance appropriations, in which VA estimates what the agency calls essential initial funding for the advance appropriations year. VA then estimates full funding for initiatives in the next year based on updated information. However, we do not address VA's approach to budgeting in this report and our recommendation is that VA state in future budget justifications whether the estimates for initiatives in support of the advance appropriations request reflect all the funding that may be required if all initiatives are continued. VA's comments indicate that all funding for these initiatives is not included in the advance appropriations estimates. VA could implement our recommendation by making a statement to this effect in its budget justification.

In addition to its comments on our recommendations, VA had comments on three sections of our report. VA questioned the accuracy of our assertion that VA did not disclose the new reporting approach for its initiatives, which included estimates for certain ongoing health care services. VA stated that a table footnote in its budget justification explained that the estimates for initiatives for fiscal years 2012, 2013, and 2014 represented total funding. We do not believe that a table footnote in a document, which consists of nearly 400 pages, provides adequate transparency in explaining a change of more than $1 billion that resulted from a new reporting approach. Moreover, because the footnote does not explain that this approach is new or that the estimate for ongoing services was also affected, we continue to believe that the transparency of VA's reporting could be improved. We support VA's plans to include an expanded narrative regarding its approach to reporting estimates for initiatives in future budget justifications and believe this will enhance transparency.

VA also indicated that it disagreed with what VA characterized as our assertion that Congress cannot use VA's estimates of costs for ongoing health care services or initiatives due to a lack of transparency. As evidence, VA pointed to the detailed information presented in the budget justification and described how the estimates are determined, including a description of the actuarial model it uses. However, we did not state that Congress cannot use VA's estimates for the cost of ongoing health care services and initiatives. Instead, what we identified was that the lack of transparency regarding the factors that changed VA's estimate for ongoing health care services and initiatives resulted in unclear information for congressional deliberation. VA's concurrence with two of our recommendations and its implementation of them would address the concerns we raised and improve the transparency of the information that VA provides to Congress in its annual budget justifications.

VA also expressed concern that our conclusions cast doubt on its strong commitment to stewardship of resources. VA noted that the agency and its resources need to be flexible and responsive to changes in veterans' medical care needs, which may occur after its budget estimates are formulated. VA has the authority to respond to such changes. We have pointed out, for example, that VA's NRM spending is consistent with its authority to increase and decrease the amounts VA allocates from the Medical Facilities account for NRM. However, in regard to NRM, the long-standing pattern in which NRM spending has significantly exceeded VA's estimates needs to be better accounted for in VA's budget estimates. Doing so will not decrease VA's flexibility to be responsive to veterans' needs. Moreover, we believe that VA's plans to address our recommendation will provide Congress with more reliable estimates with which to make decisions about VA appropriations.

We are sending copies of this report to the Secretary of Veterans Affairs and the Acting Director of the Office of Management and Budget, and appropriate congressional committees. In addition, the report will be available at no charge on the GAO website http://www.gao.gov.

If you or your staff have any questions about this report, please contact Randall B. Williamson at (202) 512-7114 or williamsonr@gao.gov, or Melissa Emrey-Arras at (617) 788-0534 or emreyarrasm@gao.gov. Contact points for our Offices of Congressional Relations and Public Affairs are on the last page of this report. GAO staff who made major contributions to this report are listed in appendix II.

Randall B. Williamson
Director, Health Care

Melissa Emrey-Arras
Acting Director, Strategic Issues

List of Committees

The Honorable Kent Conrad
Chairman
The Honorable Jeff Sessions
Ranking Member
Committee on the Budget
United States Senate

The Honorable Patty Murray
Chairman
The Honorable Richard Burr
Ranking Member
Committee on Veterans' Affairs
United States Senate

The Honorable Tim Johnson
Chairman
The Honorable Mark Kirk
Ranking Member
Subcommittee on Military Construction,
  Veterans' Affairs, and Related Agencies
Committee on Appropriations
United States Senate

The Honorable Paul Ryan
Chairman
The Honorable Chris Van Hollen
Ranking Member
Committee on the Budget
House of Representatives

The Honorable Jeff Miller
Chairman
The Honorable Bob Filner
Ranking Member
Committee on Veterans' Affairs
House of Representatives

The Honorable John Culberson
Chairman
The Honorable Sanford Bishop
Ranking Member
Subcommittee on Military Construction,
  Veterans' Affairs, and Related Agencies
Committee on Appropriations
House of Representatives

Appendix I: Comments from the Department of Veterans Affairs

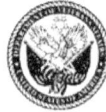

DEPARTMENT OF VETERANS AFFAIRS
WASHINGTON DC 20420
May 23, 2012

Randall Williamson
Director, Health Care
U.S. Government Accountability Office
441 G Street, NW
Washington, DC 20548

Dear Mr. Williamson:

The Department of Veterans Affairs (VA) has reviewed the Government Accountability Office's (GAO) draft report, *"VETERANS' HEALTH CARE BUDGET: Transparency and Reliability of Some Estimates Supporting President's Request Could Be Improved"* (GAO-12-689). VA concurs with two recommendations and non-concurs with one recommendation to the Department.

The enclosure specifically addresses GAO's recommendations and provides comments to the draft report. VA appreciates the opportunity to comment on your draft report.

Sincerely,

John R. Gingrich
Chief of Staff

Enclosures

Enclosure

Department of Veterans Affairs (VA) Comments to
Government Accountability Office (GAO) Draft Report:
*"VETERANS' HEALTH CARE BUDGET: Transparency and Reliability of
Some Estimates Supporting President's Request Could Be Improved"*
(GAO-12-689)

GAO Recommendation: To improve the transparency and reliability of
information presented in VA's congressional budget justifications that support
the President's budget request for VA health care, we recommend the Secretary
of VA take the following actions:

Recommendation 1: State in future budget justifications whether the estimates for
initiatives include funding for ongoing health care services.

VA Comment: Concur. VA agrees with the need for transparency. The fiscal year
2013 President's Budget included footnotes in some funding tables regarding the
display of the initiatives. In future budget justifications, VA will include a narrative
description to state whether the estimates for initiatives include funding for ongoing
health care services.

Recommendation 2: State in future budget justifications whether the estimates for
initiatives in support of the advance appropriations request reflect all the funding that
may be required if all initiatives are to be continued.

VA Comment: Non-concur. This recommendation is not consistent with the multi-year
approach to the budgeting process for advance appropriations. The purpose of
advance appropriations is to provide essential initial funding for VA's medical
appropriations to ensure continuity of health care services for Veterans. Estimates for
initiatives in support of the advance appropriations request are updated one year later in
the next President's Budget submission. The full funding that may be required if all
initiatives are to be continued would not be determined until one year after the initial
advance appropriations request is submitted.

Recommendation 3: Reflect in future budget justifications estimates of annual
resource needs for non-recurring maintenance (NRM) that fully account for resources
that VA medical facilities have consistently spent for this purpose.

VA Comment: Concur. VA will reflect in future budget justifications the annual
estimated obligations for NRM and other components of the Medical Facilities
appropriation consistent with policy decisions and past spending practices.

1

Enclosure

Department of Veterans Affairs (VA) Comments to
Government Accountability Office (GAO) Draft Report:
*"VETERANS' HEALTH CARE BUDGET: Transparency and Reliability of
Some Estimates Supporting President's Request Could Be Improved"*
(GAO-12-689)

General Comments

Page 9, paragraph 1: GAO's assertion that VA did not disclose the new reporting
approach is inaccurate. In Volume 2 of the *VA 2013 Budget Submission, Medical
Programs and Information Technology Programs*, page 1A-5, VA includes a footnote
that explains that total funding for initiatives in 2012, 2013, and 2014 appear in the
section. To further enhance transparency, VA has agreed to include an expanded
narrative in future budget submissions.

Page 11, paragraph 1: VA disagrees with GAO's claim that Congress cannot use VA
estimates for costs of ongoing healthcare or initiatives due to a lack of transparency.
The Department is committed to providing transparent and reliable budget information
to Congress. To that end, VA's budget submission provides in-depth, multi-year
analysis for health care services, with detail for specific services such as acute care,
mental health, prosthetics, and long-term care. The budget also articulates resource
needs and provides extensive details on costs of healthcare programs and initiatives
such as new facility activations, ending Veterans homelessness, and implementation of
the Caregivers Act. To develop its cost estimates for healthcare programs, VA uses a
sophisticated actuarial model, which is methodologically sound and updated annually
with revised cost, utilization, and Veteran enrollment data. VA routinely briefs
Congressional staff on the actuarial model and the data used for development of budget
requirements.

Conclusion, pages 14-15: VA is concerned that GAO's conclusion casts doubt on the
Department's strong commitment to stewardship of resources. Changes to the
Department's resource requirements are driven by changes in Veterans' medical care
needs. Shifts in mission requirements, such as the greater need for mental health
services, the need to eliminate Veteran homelessness, ensuring access to health care
for women Veterans and Veterans in rural areas – drive VA's resource requirements.
To provide the very best in compassionate and quality health care and services, VA and
its resources must be flexible and responsive to the needs of the Nation's Veterans.
It is also important to note that the level of funding included in the budget estimates for
the non-recurring maintenance (NRM) program are the result of policy decisions made
within the context of balancing the operational and capital needs of VA's healthcare
system. As with any program estimate included in the budget submission, adjustments
to the NRM program may be made in the year of execution based on emerging
operational requirements.

2

Appendix II: GAO Contacts and Staff Acknowledgments

Contacts

Randall B. Williamson, Director, Health Care, (202) 512-7114, williamsonr@gao.gov

Melissa Emrey-Arras, Acting Director, Strategic Issues, (617) 788-0534, emreyarrasm@gao.gov

Staff Acknowledgments

In addition to the contacts named above, James C. Musselwhite and Melissa Wolf, Assistant Directors; Kye Briesath, Deirdre Brown, Krister Friday, Lauren Grossman, Aaron Holling, Wati Kadzai, and Lisa Motley made key contributions to this report.

Related GAO Products

VA Health Care: Estimates of Available Budget Resources Compared with Actual Amounts. GAO-12-383R. Washington, D.C.: March 30, 2012.

VA Health Care: Methodology for Estimating and Process for Tracking Savings Need Improvement. GAO-12-305. Washington, D.C.: February 27, 2012.

Department of Veterans Affairs: Issues Related to Real Property Realignment and Future Health Care Costs. GAO-11-877T. Washington, D.C.: July 27, 2011.

Veterans' Health Care Budget Estimate: Changes Were Made in Developing the President's Budget Request for Fiscal Years 2012 and 2013. GAO-11-622. Washington, D.C.: June 14, 2011.

Veterans' Health Care: VA Uses a Projection Model to Develop Most of Its Health Care Budget Estimate to Inform the President's Budget Request. GAO-11-205. Washington, D.C.: January 31, 2011.

VA Health Care: Spending for and Provision of Prosthetic Items. GAO-10-935. Washington, D.C.: September 30, 2010.

VA Health Care: Reporting of Spending and Workload for Mental Health Services Could Be Improved. GAO-10-570. Washington, D.C.: May 28, 2010.

Continuing Resolutions: Uncertainty Limited Management Options and Increased Workload in Selected Agencies. GAO-09-879. Washington, D.C.: September 24, 2009.

VA Health Care: Challenges in Budget Formulation and Issues Surrounding the Proposal for Advance Appropriations. GAO-09-664T. Washington, D.C.: April 29, 2009.

VA Health Care: Challenges in Budget Formulation and Execution. GAO-09-459T. Washington, D.C.: March 12, 2009.

VA Health Care: Long-Term Care Strategic Planning and Budgeting Need Improvement. GAO-09-145. Washington, D.C.: January 23, 2009.

Federal Real Property: Progress Made in Reducing Unneeded Property, but VA Needs Better Information to Make Further Reductions. GAO-08-939. Washington, D.C.: September 10, 2008.

VA Health Care: Budget Formulation and Reporting on Budget Execution Need Improvement. GAO-06-958. Washington, D.C.: September 20, 2006.

www.ingramcontent.com/pod-product-compliance
Lightning Source LLC
Chambersburg PA
CBHW080937290526
45795CB00007BA/2798